The Acne-Free
30 Days to Clear

Dean R. Goodless, M.D.

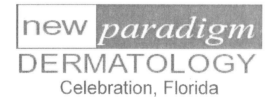

DERMATOLOGY
Celebration, Florida

ISBN Number: 1-4116-3578-7

Publisher: New Paradigm Dermatology, PL
               PO Box 470026
               Celebration, FL 34747

*Cover design by Dean, Suzi, Sebrina, Brandie,Tiffany & Nazia.
Special Thanks to Rube J. Pardo, M.D, Ph.D for reviewing the
manuscript.*

Contents

DISCLAIMER

This book is not a substitute for your physician and should not be relied upon as a source of personal medical advice. The information included herein is of a general and educational nature only and is not meant to be taken as a specific prescription for any medical condition. Vitamin, mineral and herbal supplements can have side effects and or may interfere with medications as well as pose a possible risk during pregnancy.
Please consult your physician for further guidance.

Introduction

Among the many diseases I deal with on a daily basis as a clinical and research dermatologist, acne ranks as one of the most frustrating and challenging conditions to treat. There are literally many dozens of prescription and over the counter antibiotic pills, creams and washes as well as other topical treatments that I have prescribed over the past decade, often with limited success.

A few years ago, I decided that there must be another way to deal with acne besides nearly continuous oral antibiotics and irritating and bothersome creams and cleansers. A review of the medical literature led me to a surprising realization: *There is in fact a significant body of clinical research already published which proves that many vitamins, minerals and even herbs can help clear up acne.* I was skeptical. Nonetheless, I started suggesting a combination of the most promising of these nutrients to some of my patients *instead of* oral antibiotics...*and they responded dramatically.* So much so that I founded a company to manufacture this specific combination as a nutritional supplement for people with acne – and I often recommend it to my own patients. But supplementation is not the whole story: Some foods may in fact *worsen* acne, not improve it. Thus began my quest for the ultimate nutritional solution to acne: The Acne-Free Diet Plan: *30 Days to Clearer Skin.*

1. A Pimple is Born

Sometime around puberty, and following a natural and predetermined timetable, your reproductive system begins to produce an increased amount of "male"-type hormones (yes, ladies too). These hormones are delivered throughout your body where their biochemical effects take place. Sebaceous glands in your skin respond to this stimulation with increased production of sebum, or oil. This oil is different than the existing oily substance produced by your epidermal or surface skin cells.[*] Epidermal lipids promote a healthy and normal level of desquamation of dead skin cells, keeping pores clear of debris. Sebum on the other hand, is sticky, messy oil which more or less acts like cement causing dead skin cells to plug up pores. To make matters worse, if you are genetically predisposed to acne, your sebaceous glands are *hyper-responsive* to the circulating hormones and produce so much sebum that the healthy epidermal lipids become overwhelmed and are virtually washed away by this flood of stickier oil. The result: sticky epidermal cells "glued together" by sebum form a plug at the opening of a hair follicle on your

---

[*] *Epidermal lipids are skin oils produced in and by the surface cells of the skin vs. the oil produced by sebaceous "oil" glands which are associated with every pore.*

face.   Thus   is   formed   your   first *microcomedone*:   an invisible clogged pore. Congratulations – a pimple is born.

But it doesn't end there does it? Because what was once invisible becomes clearly visible some time later, possibly as a "third eye" in the middle of your forehead. How did that happen?   Imagine that lake of oil accumulating and growing inside your newborn microcomedone. To acne bacteria, *that's good stuff. Proprionobacterium acnes* eats sebum for breakfast, lunch and dinner. And soon your little microcomedone is home to a gazillion of these guys chowing down like tourists at a buffet restaurant. And what did *P. acnes* leave behind after digesting all that delicious sebum? A very irritating substance known as free fatty acids   (FFA).   Now   your   peaceful microcomedone is starting to get a little irritated.   Some   redness,   perhaps   some swelling is noticeable. Over time, white blood cells attracted to the inflammation (like sharks to blood) begin to move in. Soon there are so many white blood cells *you can actually see them*:   a   pustule   has   formed.   You compulsively, almost instinctively, grab the offending lesion and squeeze the life out of it until…POP. Poor little pimple. Rest in peace. But before it dies it gives a final warning, in a deep, Austrian accent: *"I'll be back."*

2. The Acne-Diet Connection: Constipation to Controversy

I think it's a bit overworked – this idea that acne is a "build up of toxins" or that something: blood, liver, bowel, *whatever*, needs to be "cleansed" in order to clear up acne. Because we know now that acne is really just a genetic predisposition to a revved-up biochemical response to hormones. At least for the most part. But what did doctors think a hundred years ago? Few controlled studies were done then. There was a lot of medical *opinion* and little medical *fact*. Suffice it to say, most medical experts of the 19th century thought that *constipation* was one of the principle causative factors of acne.[1] Darier, a notable dermatologist of the era recommended *"...regular evacuation of the bowels which will sometimes have to be secured by suitable laxatives."*[2] (He also recommended bradyphagia – *eating slowly*; and *facial gymnastics* – whatever *that* is!)

But really, what about constipation and acne? And what happens to acne when you *"evacuate the bowels"* regularly? As recently as 1983, one dermatologist wrote a letter to the editor of the *Archives of Dermatology* stating:

"I believe correction of constipation is a favorable influence on acne, an opinion admittedly anecdotal, circumstantial, empirical, and tinged with folklore. I recall several highly motivated patients with acne who had a rapid, indeed almost abrupt, clearing of their acne through correction of faulty bowel elimination by means of a daily serving of 30gm of an 'all-bran' breakfast cereal."[3]

But has the idea of *fiber as a treatment for acne* been studied in a trial as suggested in this letter? No, as far as fiber and acne goes, you're on your own. But it sounds pretty low-risk and certainly harmless to try. At least your colon will thank you. Unexpectedly, these early dermatologists may have stumbled onto something. Not what they thought mind you, but something potentially useful nonetheless. Since the 1920's doctors have looked at *carbohydrates* as a possible cause of acne. And high fiber foods, being slowly digested, tend to have a low glycemic index. That is, they don't dump a lot of sugar into the bloodstream abruptly causing a spike in blood sugar and subsequently – insulin. Is this important? Probably, but more on that in chapter four.

More recently, studies have looked at whole populations (entire ethnic communities with minimal acne) and compared their diets to a typical acne-invoking western diet. There are some populations in which acne is absent: the

Kitavan islanders of Papua New Guinea and the Ache of Eastern Paraguay – both of which consume a diet which is 70% from plants.[4] South African Bantu eating a traditional plant based diet have one-third the acne of their white, western-diet fed neighbors.[4] Similar lower incidences of acne in people eating a less refined plant-based diet in countries from Europe to Japan have been noted.[5]

But *why*? What's in America's yummy burgers n' fries food pyramid that isn't in a plant-based diet and vice-versa? Beyond the high-fiber, lower glycemic index foods of Homo sapiens' traditional eats, these diets also offer *a much higher amount of omega-3 fatty acids* relative to omega-6 fatty acids as well as being nearly devoid of the dreaded, man-made, *trans* fatty acids.[6] The details of this fatty conundrum and how it relates to acne will be addressed further in chapter five where we discover why people with acne should eat more fish.

Sounds pretty convincing, so what's the controversy? Apparently, no one has yet done the proper *double-blind placebo-controlled study* on these various dietary attributes to prove a *causal* effect in regards to acne. Hence, the flurry of *letters to the editor* discounting these studies nearly just as fast as they are published. You can wait years until the "proper" studies have been done, or you can simply *connect the dots* all these retrospective and epidemiological studies lay out for you and see for yourself if you are just 30 days away from clearer skin!

3. Dietary Triggers of Acne Breakouts:
a.k.a. Every Teen's Favorite Foods

F unny how God made all the delicious food bad for you and all the (lets be honest now) less yummy food oh-so-healthy. At least God has a great a sense of humor. When you look at the roster of "foods blamed for acne", i.e. chocolate, sweets, cola, fatty foods, etc., one has to agree with Dr. Gerd Michaelsson:

> *"...this list has one remarkable feature – all of the blacklisted items are delicious and delectable for the adolescent palate."*[7]

What would this rogue's gallery of forbidden ingredients look like? Let's compile a list of suspects, and then we can put them on trial: nuts, chocolate, salt, sweets, fried foods & milk. We'll deal with milk, sweets and fried foods in depth in the chapters to come. There's also some suspicion for dietary iodine to address. But first: what did a bunch of people report as trigger foods for their acne?

Using a retrospective study more than 500 patients seen at a Taiwanese dermatology clinic over several years were surveyed.[8] There were only two dietary items that more than 30% of the respondents indicated flared their acne: *peanuts and fried food.* Capsicum (chili pepper) was blamed just over 20% of the time. Many other prime suspects were implicated *less than 10% of the time* including chocolate, cocoa, cheese, bread and cake. Poor little peanut. We'll miss you. And fried food – we'll get to you later when discussing fats. Should chocolate be let off so easily you ask? Balderdash....*heresy!?* Is it possible that *mom was wrong*? Let's take a closer look at chocolate: *the boogey man of acne trigger foods.*

Dermatology texts from the early 1900's routinely blamed chocolate as a cause of acne. But a study done in 1965 *"indicates that chocolate has been unjustly cast"* as a cause of acne.[9] Eight acne patients volunteered for this *hideous torture*, three of whom indicated previous flares of their acne from eating chocolate. They each ate nearly 20 ounces of chocolate bars over 2 days. That's something like 12 garden variety-sized chocolate bars! Up to a week later there was *no indication the chocolate had caused an acne flare* in any of the study subjects.

But the first *large* study on chocolate and acne is the oft-referenced "Fulton study".[10] Here three big name world-renowned acne experts looked at 65 acne patients with whom they *"deliberately contrived to...ingest high quantities of chocolate daily, greatly in excess of what is likely to be consumed by even the passionate lover of chocolate."* It was a single-blind study using two types of candy bars provided by a chocolate bar manufacturer.

Each bar had the same amount and types of sugars and fats but only one had chocolate added as an ingredient. It was a crossover trial which means the subjects ate one type of bar for four weeks, followed by a three week wash out period, then they ate the other type of bar for four weeks. Acne lesions were counted throughout and subjects were considered to have worsened acne if their lesion counts increased by more than 30%. Verdict: There was no statistically significant difference between acne flare ups while eating either type of bar, but *the chocolate eaters trended toward less break outs!* They then picked out four of the test subjects who had indicated prior breakouts of acne with chocolate and specifically *bombarded* them with the chocolate-containing bar to no avail: their acne did not flare. Doesn't that make you feel good! *Chocolate is innocent!* So go eat a piece of chocolate and when you come back we'll look at salt and iodine.

Let's take a quick look at salt – i.e. ordinary table salt in your salt shaker which is known technically as *sodium chloride*. An Indiana physician first noted some improvement in the acne of a patient in whom he had recommended salt restriction for blood pressure control.[11] He then took a look at the urinary *chloride* level of 30 acne patients and found it to be elevated. Finally he placed patients on a three month low sodium diet. The four patients he followed thus all showed a dramatic drop in urinary chloride with a concurrent improvement in their acne. The doctor confirmed the improvement possible in acne by applying the low salt diet *to his own self with similar results!* Such a small study offers little more than anecdotal evidence, but it's intriguing nonetheless. Especially in view of the *huge* quantities of salt typically present in a western diet. Sad that chips and salted popcorn are out? Have another piece of chocolate; it'll make you feel better.

The effects, if any, of iodine on acne are a bit more complicated to follow. Blood levels of iodine appear to be normal in acne patients and administered iodine does not seem to increase the amount of sebum produced.[12] However, *massive* quantities of iodine can cause an *acne-like* eruption.[13] Worsening or development of acne has been reported in patients taking multiple *Kelp* tablets (containing 15mg of iodine each).[14] For this reason, some dermatologists have recommended restriction of *iodized* salt and or *seafood* for acne sufferers. But can the iodine content of *food* influence the severity of *acne vulgaris*? One large epidemiological survey examined the dietary habits of over 1000 students in North Carolina.[15] So many assumptions were made and the statistical analysis so convoluted that interpretation of the results is tricky. Although no difference was seen in the incidence of acne based upon iodine intake, it was noted that the principle sources of dietary iodine were *iodized salt* and *water* with food *including seafood* minimally impacting. It seems unlikely the amounts of iodine normally found in *food* affects acne.

4. Cows, Carbs and Hormones

Everyone knows sweets cause acne right? Soda, candy, cookies, and sugary foods are near the top of the acne trigger foods hit list. *But should they be?* What does the literature tell us about glucose metabolism in people with acne and the effects of altering carbohydrate intake on the severity of acne? More interesting still, what about altering the carbohydrate metabolism itself? And what's all this commotion about milk and acne? We don't think of milk as a sweet or high glycemic index food, and it really doesn't rocket blood glucose up like a sweet. But it *does* rocket *insulin* up as if it were a sugar load.[16] Insulin...that's a hormone, right? And we all know that *hormones are the root of all pimples.* No argument there. So let's see if we can link these three together in some sort sinister relationship with acne: Cows, carbs and hormones.

Glucose tolerance *per se* in acne patients appears to be normal, and limiting sugar does not appear to be an effective treatment for the disease.[17] But there's definitely something afoot here. More than 50% of acne patients in one study had fasting hyperglycemia, though not overtly diabetic.[18] And glucose metabolism was disturbed in 80% of female acne patients during the peri-menstrual period, a time when many women complain of acne flare-ups.[19] At the hormonal level, a high carb diet (vs. a high protein one) tends to shunt circulating testosterone to the acne-causing *dihydrotestosterone* form.[20]

What about glucose metabolism in the skin itself, the concept of "skin diabetes"?[21] *Blood* glucose tolerance curves may be normal in acne, but glucose removal from the *skin* is delayed compared to healthy controls.[22] And here is where things really get interesting: Non-diabetic acne patients treated with oral medications for diabetes show improvement in their skin.[23,24]

The overall picture then *vis-à-vis* glucose metabolism and acne seems best summed up by Mullins and Naylor who state:

> *No amount of avoidance of high carbohydrate foods will save those with a marked genetically determined susceptibility; nor will massive amounts of cutaneous sugar affect those without the genetically prepared skin. Between these extremes lies the major portion of our acne patients. In this middle group excessive or repeated blood glucose elevations will definitely raise the average amount of glucose present in the skin per unit time and we feel this will definitely produce a greater total number of (acne lesions).[25]*

But even if *skin diabetes* exists, what is the mechanism by which it can promote acne? In other words, how does eating more carbs in a person predisposed to problems with carbohydrate metabolism cause pimples? For the answer, let's look at another disease.

Polycystic Ovary Syndrome is a condition where hormone-producing ovarian cysts produce excess "male" hormones such as dehydroepiandrosterone sulfate (DHEAS) and dihydrotestosterone (DHT). This results in a triad of obesity, excess facial hair and *acne*. Also in this condition, there is *insensitivity to insulin*. Insulin is the hormone your body uses to handle blood glucose levels after you've ingested a load of carbohydrates. When blood glucose can't be kept in check with insulin due to *insulin resistance*, the body compensates by increasing insulin production. Most important for us, as insulin is increased a closely related hormone called *insulin-like growth factor* (IGF-1) is also increased. PCOS then gives us a valuable clue in figuring out how carbs can cause acne: dietary carbs cause insulin to go up (even more so in PCOS due to insulin resistance) and IGF-1 follows insulin's lead. The IGF-1 and ovarian hormones appear to act in concert to promote acne. This biological "dance" between IGF-1 and the acne-causing hormones DHEAS and DHT has been studied.[26] It seems that elevated levels of these two "male" hormones stimulate acne only when IGF-1 levels are elevated. In other words, IGF-1 is the *facilitator*, allowing the increased hormones to cause acne. And when are these hormones typically increased? You guessed it – at puberty and around the middle of the menstrual cycle.

But back to common everyday acne: are IGF-1 levels elevated in *acne vulgaris*? One recent study indicated they are.[27] And two others demonstrated not just elevated IGF-1 in adult women with acne, but insulin resistance as well.[28,29]

But what is it about IGF-1 that causes acne? When the effect of IGF-1 on sebaceous gland cells was studied this hormone was found to be *the most potent stimulus to the growth of these cells*, thereby increasing sebum production in concert with other hormones.[30] Cordain[4] elegantly reviewed several mechanisms whereby IGF-1 may cause acne including: directly causing proliferation of keratinocytes which can clog pores; indirectly influencing the retinoid receptors[*] in cells thereby inhibiting normal maturation and shedding of keratinocytes; and stimulating not just enhanced production of "male" hormones but inhibiting the production of *sex hormone binding globulin* (SHBG) whose job it is to keep those hormones bound-up and inactivated (think of SHBG as a kind of circulating sponge designed by nature to soak up excess hormones in the blood). It's no surprise then that *injecting IGF-1 into humans causes outbreaks of acne.*[31] IGF-1...*Bad!*

It may be worthwhile to recall that milk, like carbohydrate, increases IGF-1 (about 10% above baseline).[32] But does milk cause acne?

---

[*] *Retinoid receptors are activated by vitamin A as well as drugs such as Retin-A® or Accutane®, and are responsible for normal skin cell maturation and exfoliation.*

After all, milk is absent from the Kitavan and Ache indigenous diets (just as acne is absent from their skin).[4]

The Nurses Health Study II is an ongoing prospective study designed to look at lifestyle and disease correlations. Over 45,000 women in this study were surveyed regarding their milk intake and incidence of teenage acne and *a positive association* was found.[33] A positive association was also found for vitamin D *from supplements*. The authors implicated hormones as the factor in milk that made acne worse. Not just the androgenic hormones *within* the milk and the IGF-1 it *contains* and apparently *stimulates*, but the *body's altered handling of testosterone* as a result of vitamin D supplementation.

In summary, there is evidence which implicates an abnormality of carbohydrate metabolism (insulin resistance) as a factor in acne. Some of the data implies that dietary intake of carbohydrates in genetically predisposed persons with insulin resistance may be the unlucky combination that results in acne, possibly by increasing IGF-1 at a time (puberty or mid-menstrual cycle) when "male" hormones (DHEAS, DHT or progesterone[*]) are increased. Consuming large quantities of milk may also be undesirable in people prone to acne since it too raises IGF-1 and two groups studied who drink no milk also have no acne.

---

[*] *Progesterone is an androgenic ("male") hormone released mid-menstrual cycle which causes ovulation – the release of an egg from the ovary.*

The evidence between carbohydrates and acne seems most compelling for adult women with post-adolescent acne, but may be helpful to others as well.

5. Good Fats, Bad Fats: Fish Don't Get Pimples

Without getting too much into the biochemistry involved, dietary fats differ in their effects upon the body. Some dietary fats contain a portion or fatty acid known as "omega 3" and others known as "omega 6". There are others, but these are the two groups I am going to harass you with for now. Also know that there is an *evil* fat known as "trans" fat which is essentially man-made. It was originally designed to replace butter as a fat that wouldn't go rancid. As you can imagine, if even bacteria won't have it, you probably shouldn't either. So let's look at where these fats come from and how they affect your body, especially in regards to possible effects on acne.

It is believed that man's early diet consisted of a balance of omega-3 vs. omega-6 oils, i.e. a 1:1 ratio. [34] The modern western diet warps this ratio dramatically to something like a 20:1 ratio of omega-6 to omega-3. And why does this matter? It seems that omega-6 fatty acids are metabolized by the body in such a way as to increase pro-inflammatory chemicals like leukotriene B_4 (LTB$_4$ for short). These chemicals appear to be intimately involved in the development of acne. For example, if you treat people experimentally with a chemical that blocks the activity of LTB_4, their acne improves.[35] So are omega-3 oils any better? *Yes, by far.* Firstly, omega-3 oils are metabolized into *anti-inflammat*ory chemicals (not pro-inflammatory like omega-6); and secondly, omega-3 oils can increase a useful molecule *called insulin-like growth factor binding protein-3.*[36] This chemical is like nature's sponge for soaking up IGF-1, and if you remember...IGF-1 = *bad.* So anything that reduces IGF-1 must be good, at least as far as acne is concerned. And that evil "trans" fat? It is also metabolized into pro-inflammatory chemicals.[37]

Is there any evidence that you can manipulate the sebum itself, either its makeup or its volume, by altering the diet? Doubtful. The oils you eat are *not* excreted unchanged in sebum:

> *It is unlikely that dietary lipids are excreted unchanged in sebum or that a modest increase in ingested lipids results in an increase in sebum excretion rate.*[38]

However, *fasting* will result in a reduction in sebum production after about 5 days.[39] Obviously, fasting is only a short term option. Even a prolonged low fat diet does not improve acne unless you then supplement the diet with *unsaturated fat.*[40] In that case there is considerable improvement in acne.

18

So what about fish and why don't fish get pimples? Easy – they're *loaded* with omega-3's. Well that, plus they don't have any pores. But fish are only one source of omega-3's. Omega-3 fats can be found in both plant and animal sources. Animal sources are for the most part cold water fish, with wild game like venison or buffalo also being reasonable sources. There are many plant sources of omega-3 fats with flax oil being far and away the best plant source of omega-3 oils. For the most part, other meats and eggs are loaded with omega-6 oils.

In order to get the desired effect from your intake of omega-3 oils, you should try to limit your intake of omega-6 oils. Remember that a typical western diet has an omega-6:omega-3 ratio of up to 20:1. The closer you can bring this to a 1:1 ratio of the hunter/gatherer diet (human beings' evolutionarily correct diet), the better. Its difficult to cook with omega-3's because when heated they become evil *trans* fats. And you'll want to avoid using too much omega-6's as your cooking oil. So rely on Olive oil as your good all around work horse oil. Olive oil is a mono-unsaturated oil and is "inflammatory neutral". So in summary: eat a low fat diet, using Olive oil as your principle fat, avoiding trans-fats altogether, and supplementing with omega-3 oils to help bring you closer to a 1:1 ratio with omega-6's.

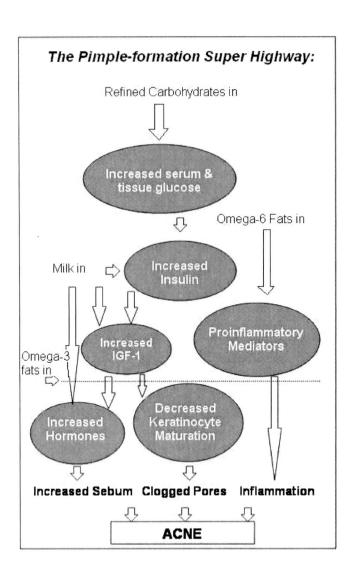

6. Vitamins, Minerals and Surprising Clinical Studies

This being the original subject of my look at non-medicinal treatments for acne is sort of like the meat n' potatoes part of this book. I first started looking at nutritional supplements for acne a few years back and was surprised to find numerous clinical studies had already been done which showed benefit in acne from using certain vitamins and minerals. I then packaged the most promising of these into a combination packet and tried it in a few of my patients, and they liked it. *They liked it so much, they asked if they could buy it.* And so Skinutrients™ was born. Skinutrients markets a nutritional supplement for acne called Accunatural™ which contains most of the vitamins and minerals discussed in this chapter in a convenient three-tablet formula. You could also purchase any of the vitamins mentioned here at your local health food store and make up your own anti-acne packets.

Vitamin A:
There are very few studies involving vitamin A alone in acne (usually using huge doses) however studies with both vitamin A *and* zinc have demonstrated no additional benefit by the addition of vitamin A in doses as high as 200,000IU daily, a clearly toxic dose.[41,42] The RDA for vitamin A in adolescent

and adult males (the highest RDA for humans) is 3000IU. The Food and Nutrition Board (FNB) of the Institute of Medicine has set the *tolerable upper level of intake* of vitamin A at 10000IU per day with higher levels raising concerns re: osteoporosis. Based upon all the data and concerns regarding toxicity of higher doses of vitamin A it seems prudent to keep the supplemental dosage in the 3000IU to 10000IU range as a measure to avoid deficiency and to maximize bioavailability as well as long term safety.

Vitamin B5:

A Hong-Kong based researcher felt that pantothenic acid (vitamin B5) could play a role in acne. He theorized that around puberty, the body shifts the utilization of pantothenic acid, an important co-enzyme, from fatty acid metabolism toward steroid synthesis (to produce increased hormones). The resulting decrease in normal fatty acid metabolism could lead to acne. By supplementing with large doses of pantothenic acid, this relative deficiency could be removed and acne improved. He tested his theory in 100 Asian patients at doses as high as 10gm of pantothenic acid per day tapering to a maintenance dose of 1gm per day as allowed by improvement in acne and reported that the treatment was effective.[43] There is little toxicity noted from mega-doses of B5, even up to 20gm per day.

Vitamin B6:

An early study showed benefits of pyridoxine (vitamin B6) in treatment-resistant acne.[44] There was support shown specifically for pre-menstrual flare up of acne in another published study where 106 young women with documented pre-menstrual flare ups of their acne were given 50mg daily of vitamin B6 and a statistically significant improvement was documented.[45] The mechanism for this improvement is not known, however it may involve *normalization* of testosterone uptake and sensitivity in target tissues.[46] Before using mega-dose B6 for acne, be certain *that acne vulgaris* is the diagnosis and not *rosacea* (sometimes called adult acne) because the latter can be aggravated by high doses of B6.[47]

Zinc:

There are so many studies on the effectiveness of zinc for acne that they will not be reviewed here except to say *that zinc works great in inflammatory acne*, as well as tetracycline in fact.[48,49,50,51] One problem with oral zinc, especially zinc sulphate, is that it is an *emetic* (makes you puke) so that high doses tend to be poorly tolerated. A useful question then might be *how little zinc does it take to improve acne*? And the answer would be *as little as 30mg a day* of elemental zinc.[52] Another concern with zinc supplementation is the fact *that zinc competes with copper* for absorption from the intestine. So supplementing with too much zinc over the long term could cause *copper deficiency*. A second useful question then would be *how much zinc can you take without having to worry about copper deficiency?* The answer to this question is 50mg per day. Hence somewhere between 30-50mg per day of elemental zinc would be a good reference point for using zinc as an acne-fighting supplement. Better still: OptiZinc® is InterHealth's original methionine-bound zinc ingredient which does *not* interfere with copper absorption.

Vitamin E and Selenium:
Some acne patients have decreased blood selenium levels and decreased glutathione peroxidase (an important selenium-dependant anti-oxidant enzyme).[53] Treatment of these patients for 6-12 weeks with supplemental selenium and tocopheryl succinate (dry vitamin E) restored their glutathione peroxidase levels and improved their acne as well.[54]

Chromium:
Chromium is an important nutritional co-factor necessary for normal glucose metabolism, likely by enhancing insulin sensitivity, something which may be a problem in acne.[28] Based upon the above, can supplementing with chromium improve acne? Treatment using a form of yeast with especially high chromium content did help ten patients with acne in one small study.[55]

Multivitamin Combinations:

A comprehensive plan to treat acne which included vitamin A, vitamin E, vitamin B-6, using benzoyl peroxide 5% gel nightly, and eating a well balanced, low fat, low sugar diet was studied. The subjects avoided iron and iron-fortified foods, birth control pills or hormones, iodine and iodized salt, soft drinks (which may contain brominated vegetable oils – bromine like iodine may cause acne), milk, and vitamin B-12. *Ninety percent of the patients had a good to excellent response.*[56]

Another study looked at a combination of vitamins A, B6, E, pantothenic acid, zinc, selenium and chromium along with Barberry root bark powder (a source of berberine – discussed in the next chapter). Seven patients completed the study, which showed a 50% reduction in both inflammatory and non-inflammatory (clogged pores) lesions over 30 days.[57] No other dietary manipulations or restrictions were implemented but it would be interesting to see if these results could be even better in the setting of specific dietary guidelines.

7. Looking East: Herbal Acne Therapies of India, China and Japan

Traditional medicine is based on theories of disease causes and treatments totally different than Western medicine. Most of the treatments were more or less discovered by trial and error over many centuries. In this manner some of these traditions have fortuitously stumbled upon herbal treatments for acne that actually work. The interesting part is finding out *why*.

For example, traditional Chinese medicine (TCM) and traditional Japanese medicine (Kampo) both have herbal concoctions for acne that have beneficial effects. [58,59,60] Scientists in these countries are in the process of working backwards, i.e. dissecting these multi-herbal formulations to try and find which compounds and chemicals are the ones that are having the beneficial effects. Most Kampo formulations for acne use herbs such as *Coptidis rhizoma*, *Phellodendron* bark, *Scutellaria* root and others. The common denominator among these herbs is their high content of *berberine*, an alkaloid compound known for its antiseptic and antibacterial qualities in traditional medicine. When scientists studied berberine *in-vitro* (in a test tube or culture dish) they discovered three distinct anti-acne qualities. Firstly, berberine inhibits the growth of *Proprionobacterium acnes*; secondly it inhibits the enzyme *P. acnes* uses (lipase) to generate those irritating free fatty acids that cause pimples to get red; lastly, berberine inhibits the production of oil by sebocytes, the cells lining the sebaceous gland.[61,62] Is it any wonder these herbal remedies have a beneficial effect on acne?

In India, another form of traditional medicine called Ayurvedic medicine is widely practiced. Here again, there are some herbal formulations which have shown benefit for acne patients in clinical trials.[63] In one trial, an herbal formulation called *Sunder Vati* reduced inflammatory acne lesions by 60% over 6 weeks in a double-blind randomized placebo-controlled clinical trial.[64] Non-inflammatory lesions were reduced to a lesser, but still substantial degree. The herbs used in the formulation tested comprised *Holarrhena antidysenterica, Emblica officinalis, Embelia ribes*, and *Zingiber officinale*. The mechanism of action of these herbs has not been elucidated, but was proposed to have something to do with vitamin C content, immunomodulatory activity, antibacterial activity, and anti-inflammatory activity.

Another Ayurvedic herb, Gugul *(Commiphora mukul* - known in the west as the biblical herb *Myrrh*) was tested against acne with the commonly used acne antibiotic *tetracycline* used as a control.[65] There was no statistically significant difference between the two treatments, with the herbal medicine producing a 68% reduction in inflammatory lesions over 3 months – especially in subjects with oily skin to start. The principle component of *C. mukul* believed to improve acne is *gugulipid* a compound which, like *berberine*, inhibits bacterial lipases resulting in fewer free fatty acids and subsequent inflammation.[66]

8. Other Acne Triggers: Separating Urban Myths from Scientific Fact

Washing

Mom always said you got acne because "you don't wash your face enough"![67]   But could mom *once again* be wrong?   An unpublished study looked at washing with a mild cleanser once, twice or four times daily. It appeared that twice daily washing was optimal.[68]   Washing too much is generally believed to cause irritation, and in fact, some soap components may be comedogenic - both factors likely contribute to worsening of acne.[69] And remember those "sandy" soaps that used to be so popular – liquid soap with small grains designed to *abrade away* clogged pores and acne? Well that gritty stuff added to the soap doesn't do a thing to improve acne.[70]   I generally recommend a mild soap-free liquid cleanser for my acne patients, or if they prefer, a mild wash with benzoyl peroxide or salicylic acid added.

Sunlight

Let's shine a little light on the subject of light and acne. It's interesting to note that a new treatment modality known as "blue light" therapy was recently approved by the FDA and is currently available at many dermatologists' offices.   The studies show some people definitely improve with this treatment, but not all.   In the past, a quartz light generating ultraviolet waves was used to induce peeling and treat acne. Are we going "back to the future" with blue light treatment? Not really. Blue (visible) light is *not* ultraviolet (invisible) light. Nor does blue light have any risks such as burning or skin cancer which are two likely reasons the quartz light treatment for acne went bye bye. But does ultraviolet light help acne anyway? Probably not. About 3% of patients with acne experience worsening when exposed to sunlight, a problem which is ameliorated with the use of sunscreen.[71] It appears that *squalene*, a principle component of skin oils becomes comedogenic (clogs pores) when exposed to ultraviolet radiation.[72]

Stress

Stress isn't likely a root cause of acne – but it certainly doesn't *help* any rash that I know of (including acne). That being said, what data is there regarding stress and acne? In Yeh's survey of Taiwanese acne patients, stress, insufficient sleep and combination of the above were notable acne trigger factors independent of school examination periods which were a negligible influence.[8] A more recent study using a prospective design and an objective psychological measure of stress showed that both increased perceived stress and increased acne occurred at times of school examinations.[73] In the latter study, there was a trend toward decreased sleep aggravating acne - but this didn't reach statistical significance. Diminished insulin sensitivity due to lack of sleep may be playing a role here.[74]

9. Putting it All Together: Clearer Skin in Thirty days

So here it is in a nutshell: everything that's been shown to help acne: diet, nutrition, and lifestyle-wise. What to eat, what to do, what not to do, and what nutritional supplements to take. Your goal should be noticeably clearer skin within thirty days with continued improvement thereafter. Remember that inflammatory acne lesions often leave flat pink or dark marks behind which can take 3-6 months to fade – don't worry about these, they *will* fade naturally. Judge your progress on the number of *new* raised red pimples, pustules and clogged pores you are averaging week by week, month by month. A decreasing trend over time means improvement! Carry on until your goal is met and good luck!

Tip #1: Eat fiber everyday - Dr. Darier will be proud and your colon will be happy!

Tip #2: Avoid peanuts and fried foods – 500 Taiwanese can't be all wrong!

Tip #3: Minimize salt – avoid table salt (especially iodized), canned foods, lunch meats, chips, etc. that have excess salt.

Tip #4: Avoid milk and dairy products – soy milk may be better, it has a mix of omega-3 and omega-6 oils, just avoid brands with added sugars.

Tip # 5: Avoid *high glycemic index* foods – eat only unprocessed complex carbohydrates such as veggies and some fruits. No sodas, cakes, cookies or candies (see appendix for tables).

Tip #6: Eat a low fat diet, using principally olive oil for cooking. Minimize omega-6 oils and actually supplement with omega-3 oils to bring the ratio of these two as close to 1:1 as possible – think *caveman* (see appendix for tables).

Tip # 7: Take vitamin and mineral supplements, specifically vitamin A, vitamin E, vitamin B6, pantothenic acid, zinc, chromium and selenium (see appendix for tables).

Tip #9: Consider herbal therapies such as *berberine* containing herbs or *Ayurvedic* herbs (see appendix for suggestions).

Tip # 10: Wash twice daily with a mild non-abrasive cleanser – no more, no less. I like a soap-free liquid cleanser most of the time but you can use a wash with salicylic acid if your face is very oily or you have many clogged pores or you can use a mild benzoyl peroxide cleanser if you have a lot of red papules and pustules. You can even alternate the two types of medicated cleansers if you have the whole kit and caboodle: clogged pores, red pimples and white pustules.

Tip # 11: Use a sunscreen – oil free and non-comedogenic *please*. You'll not only avoid acne, you'll avoid wrinkles too – *bonus!*

Tip # 12: Minimize the *effects* of stress. You can't actually minimize stress – it's a part of life. But you can plan ahead. Make an effort to get your normal sleep time in during exam or stressful periods. Try to maintain your routine i.e. bedtimes, exercise, mealtimes, etc. to minimize the effects of the stressful event.

Tip # 13: Be aware of the way foods affect your skin – stay off *"the pimple-formation superhighway"!*

10. Appendix

Eating Like a Hunter-Gatherer:
The glycemic *index* (GI) measures a food's ability to raise your blood glucose, and hence insulin (and therefore IGF-1 = *bad*). The glycemic *load* (GL) is a measure of just how much damage a 100g (roughly 4oz) portion of that particular food can do. In both cases, *lower is better.* When eating foods with a higher glycemic index, minimize portion size to keep the glycemic load within reason.

Refined Foods (some are ®)			Traditional Foods		
Food	GI	GL	Food	GI	GL
Rice cereal	88	77	Baked potato	85	18
Jelly beans	80	74	Boiled millet	71	17
Corn flakes	84	73	Boiled broad beans	79	15
Hard candies	70	68	Boiled couscous	65	15
Rice cakes	82	67	Boiled sweet potato	54	13
Table sugar	65	65	Boiled brown rice	55	13
Shredded wheat	69	57	Banana	53	12
Graham crackers	74	57	Boiled yam	51	12
Grape nuts	67	54	Garbanzo beans	33	9
Cheerios	74	54	Pineapple	66	8
Rye crisps	65	54	Grapes	43	8
Vanilla wafers	77	50	Kiwi	52	7
Corn chips	73	46	Carrots	71	7
Mars bar	68	42	Peas	48	7
Wheat thins	67	42	Beets	64	6
Granola bar	61	40	Kidney beans	27	6
Angel food cake	67	39	Apple	39	6
Bagel	72	38	Lentils	29	6
Doughnuts	76	38	Pear	36	5
White bread	70	35	Watermelon	72	5
Waffles	76	34	Orange	43	5
All-Bran	42	32	Cherries	22	4
Whole wheat bread	69	32	Peach	28	3
Croissant	67	31	Peanuts	14	3

Omega-3 oils are metabolized into non-inflammatory factors while omega-6 oils are metabolized into pro-inflammatory factors. Monounsaturated oils like olive oil are neutral in this regard, and can be used for cooking, unlike most omega-3 oils. A good way to supplement your daily intake of omega-3 oils is a portion of walnuts, 1-2 teaspoons of flax seed oil or a serving of salmon. Flaxseed oil can be mixed cold into salad dressing or a smoothie, but it can only be added to cooked food *after* cooking and never heated above 160°C. Trans-fats are also metabolized into pro-inflammatory factors and should be avoided.

Plant Ω-3 oil	Animal Ω-3 oil	Ω-6 oil	Trans-fat
Flax seed oil	Salmon	Borage oil	Shortening
Flax seeds	Tuna	Corn oil	Margarine
Hemp oil	Mackerel	Peanut oil	Fried fast foods
Rapeseed oil	Herring	Primrose oil	Hydrogenated
Pumpkin seed	Trout	Safflower oil	vegetable oils*
walnuts	King crab	Sesame oil	
Canola oil	Shrimp	Sunflower oil	
	Cod		
	Venison		
	Buffalo		

*hydrogenated and partially hydrogenated vegetable oils are found in most packaged snack foods such as crackers, cookies, cakes, pastries, snack foods and frozen convenience foods – for the most part *cavemen didn't eat these*.

Which Vitamins and Minerals Should You Take?:

Consider taking any of the following vitamins and minerals for their proven beneficial effect on acne:

Nutrient	Total Daily Dose
Vitamin A	3000IU-10000IU
Vitamin E	200-400IU
Vitamin B-6	50mg
Pantothenic acid	500mg-1000mg
Zinc (OptiZinc® brand)	30-50mg
Selenium	200 micrograms
Chromium (Chromate® brand)	200-400 micrograms

Which Herbs Should You Consider?:

Traditional Chinese Medicine formulations with *Coptidis rhyzoma* or the Japanese Kampo formula no. TJ-50 known as *keigai-rengyo-to* have herbs with a high berberine content, useful for fighting acne. Other herbs more commonly used in the west including Barberry (*Berberis vulgaris*), Goldenseal *(Hydrastasis canandensis)* and Oregon *grape (Berberis aquifolium)* also contain high quantities of berberine.

The Ayurvedic herb Gugul is apparently as effective as tetracycline in fighting acne – especially in those with oily skin. The Ayurvedic Medicine formula known as Sunder Vati includes four herbs. The components of the individual tablets are:

Herb	Part	mg/tablet
Holarrhena antidysenterica	Stem bark	180mg
Emblica officinalis	Dried fruit	30mg
Embelia ribes	Dried fruit	30mg
Zingiber officinale	Rhizome	10mg

The study dosage used was two 250mg tablets three times daily after meals.

Where Can You Find the Vitamins, Minerals & Herbs?:

Looking for berberine? HUANG LIAN SU contains 100% *Coptidis Rhyzoma* in the form of tea tablets (Chinese patent medicine). Easily found at your local Chinese grocery if they stock patent meds (most do), or do a Google® search for "huang lian su" good for about 300 or more hits. It's traditionally used for diarrhea (there's that pesky colon again). You won't have as much luck looking for the Kampo formula TJ-50: it's only available in Japan! Barberry and Goldenseal are readily available on line or at your neighborhood health food store where you can also assemble *"the magnificent 7"*: the vitamins and minerals mentioned above. Now I know what you're thinking: "Why doesn't someone just put all the good stuff in one tablet". Well, you're in luck. Go to www.skinutrients.com for a multi-vitamin/multi-mineral formulation which also contains Barberry as a source of berberine – *Huzzah*! If you're going to supplement with flaxseed oil, buy the refrigerated kind in the brown (light-protected) bottle. For safe and pure omega-3 from a fish, try OmegaRx® from www.zonelabsinc.com. Unfortunately, there's no commercially available *Sunder Vati* supplement, but an Ayurvedic practitioner could probably whip some up for you. Guggul on the other hand is readily available either online or at your local health food store. Check for *guggulsterone* content – the dose studied provided 25mg of guggulsterone twice daily.

11. References

[1] Bateman, T. A Practical Synopsis of Cutaneous Diseases. 8th Ed. London, Longman, Rees, Orme, Brown, Green and Longman, 1836. P. 333

[2] Darier, J. A Text-book of Dermatology. Philadelphia. Lea & Febiger, 1920. P 388

[3] Kaufman W. The Diet and Acne [letter]. Arch Derm 1983: 276

[4] Cordain L, Lindeberg S, Hurtado M, Hill K, Eaton SB, Brand-Miller J. Acne vulgaris: a disease of Western civilization. Arch Dermatol. 2002;138:1584-1590

[5] Hoehn GH. Acne and Diet. Cutis. 1966;2:389-94

[6] Cordain L In Reply [letter] Arch Dermatol 2003;139:942-43

[7] Michaelsson G. Diet and acne. Nutr Rev 1981;39(2):104-106

[8] Yeh H-P. Acne in Taiwan. J Formosan Med Assoc 1975;74:212-219

[9] Grant JD, Anderson PC. Chocolate as a cause of acne: A dissenting view. Mo Med 1965;62:459-60

[10] Fulton JE, Plewig G, Kligman AM. Effect of chocolate on acne vulgaris. JAMA 1969;210:2071-2074

[11] Gaul LE. Salt restriction in acne vulgaris. J Indiana State Med Assoc 1965;58:839-42

[12] Traub EF, Emmett R. Blood iodine of patients with acne vulgaris. Arch Dermatol Syphilol 1940;41:506

[13] Sulzberger MB, Rostenberg A, Sher JJ. Acneform eruptions with remarks on acne vulgaris and its pathogenesis. NY J med 1934

[14] Harrell BL, Rudolph AH. Kelp Diet: A Cause of Acneiform Eruption. Arch Derm 1976;112: 560

[15] Hitch JM, Greenburg BG. Adolescent acne and dietary iodine. Arch Dermatol 1961;898:911

[16] Ostman EM, Liljenberg E, Imstahl HG, Bjorck IM. Inconsistency between glycemic and insulinemic responses to regular and fermented milk products. Am J Clin Nutr 2001;74:96-100

[17] Cornbleet T, Gigli I. Should we limit sugar in acne? Arch Dermatol 1961;83:968

[18] Levin OL, Kahn M. Biochemical studies in diseases of the skin. II Acne vulgaris. Am J M Sc 1922;164:379-385

[19] Semon HC, Herrmann FS. Sugar metabolism and insulin therapy in acne vulgaris. Proc Roy Soc Med 1939;32-3:1399-1402

[20] Kappas A, Anderson KE, Conney AH, Pantuck EJ, Fishman J, Bradlow HL. Nutrition-endocrine interactions: induction of reciprocal changes in the delta-5-alpha-reduction of testosterone and the cytochrome P-450-dependent oxidation of estradiol by dietary macronutrients in man. Proc Natl Acad Sci USA 1983;80:7646-9

[21] Urbach E, Lentz JW. Carbohydrate metabolism and the skin. AMA Arch Derm Syph 1945;52:301-316

[22] Abdel KM, El Mofty A, Ismail A, Bassili F. Glucose tolerance in blood and skin of patients with acne vulgaris. Ind J Dermatol 1977;22:139-49

[23] Cohen J, Cohen A. Pustular acne staphyloderma and its treatment with tolbutamide. Can Med Assoc J. 1959; 80:629-32

[24] McIntyre DR, Johnson JA, Fusaro RM. Cutaneous extracellular glucose kinetics in acne patients receiving phenformin. Ann NY Acad Sci 1968;148(3):833-9

[25] Mullins JF, Naylor D. Glucose and the acne diathesis: an hypothesis and review of pertinent literature. Tex Rep Biol Med 1962;20:161-75

[26] Cappel M, Mauger D, Thiboutot D. Correlation between serum levels of insulin-like growth factor 1, dehydroepiandrosterone sulfate, and dihydrotestosterone and acne lesion counts in adult women. Arch Dermatol 1005;141:333-38

[27] Thiboutot D, Gilliland K, Light J, Lookingbill D. Androgen metabolism in sebaceous glands from subjects with and without acne. Arch Dermatol 1999;135:1041-5

[28] Aizawa H, Niimura M. Elevated serum insulin-like growth factor-1 (IGF-1) levels in women with postadolescent acne. J Dermatol 1995;22:249-252

[29] Aizawa H, Niimura M. Mild insulin resistance during oral glucose tolerance test (OGTT) in women with acne. J Dermatol 1996;23:526-529

[30] Deplewski D, Rosenfield RL. Growth hormone and insulin-like growth factors have

different effects on sebaceous cell growth and differentiation. Endocrinology. 1999 Sep;140(9):4089-94.

[31] Klinger B, Anin S, Silbergeld A, Eshet R, Laron Z. Development of hyperandrogenism during treatment with insulin-like growth hormone factor-1 (IGF-1) in female patients with Laron syndrome. Clin Endocrinol 1998;48:81-87

[32] Heaney RP, McCarron DA, Dawson-Hughes B, Oparil S, Berga SL, Stern JS, Barr SI, Rosen CJ. Dietary changes favorably affect bone remodeling in older adults. J Am Dietetic Asso 1999;99:1228-33

[33] Adebamowo CA, Spiegelman D, Danby FW, Frazier AL, Willett WC, Holmes MD. High school dietary dairy intake and teenage acne. J Am Acad Dermatol 2005;52:207-14

[34] Simopoulos AP, Evolutionary aspects of diet and essential fatty acids. World Rev Nutr Diet 2001;88:18-27

[35] Zouboulis CC. Is acne vulgaris a genuine inflammatory disease? Dermatology 2001;203:277-279

[36] SJ Bhathena, E Berlin, JT Judd, YC Kim, JS Law, HN Bhagavan, R Ballard-Barbash and PP Nair. Effects of omega 3 fatty acids and vitamin E on hormones involved in carbohydrate and lipid metabolism in men. Am J Clin Nutr 1991;54:684-688

[37] Calder PC. Dietary modification of inflammation with lipids. Proc Nutr Soc 2002;61:345-358

[38] Rasmussen JE. Diet and acne. Int J dermatol 1977;16:488-92

[39] Pochi PE, Downing DT, Strauss JS. Sebaceous gland resopnse in man to prolonged total caloric deprivation. J Invest Dermatol 1970;55:308

[40] Hubler WR. Unsaturated fatty acids in acne. Arch Dermatol 1959;79:644

[41] Kligman AM, Mills TH, Leyden JJ, Gross PR, Allen HB, Rudolph RI. Oral Vitamin A in Acne Vulgaris: Preliminary report. Int. J Dermatol 1981;20:278-285

[42] Michaelsson G, Juhlin L, Vahlquist A. Effects of oral zinc and vitamin A in acne. Arch Dermatol 1977;113:31-36

[43] Leung LH. Pantothenic acid deficiency as the pathogenesis of acne vulgaris. Medical Hypotheses 1995;44;490-92

[44] Joliffe N, Rosenblum LA, Sawhill J. Effects of pyridoxine (vit B6) on resistant adolescent acne. J Invest Dermatol 1941;5:143-8

[45] Snider BL, Dieteman DF. Pyridoxine therapy for premenstrual acne flare. Arch Dermatol 1974;110:130-1

[46] Symes E, Bender D, Bowen J, Coulson W. Increased target tissue uptake of, and sensitivity to, testosterone in the vitamin-B6-deficient rat. J Steroid Biochem 1984;20:1089-93

[47] Sheretz EF. Acneiform eruption due to "megadose" vitamins B6 and B12. Cutis 1991;48:119-20

[48] Hillstrom L, Pettersson L, Hellbe L, Kjellin A, Leczinsky C-G, Nordwall C. Comparison of oral treatment with zinc sulphate and placebo in acne vulgaris Br J Dermatol 1977;97:681-684

[49] Verma KC, Saini AS, Dhamija SK. Oral zinc sulphate therapy in acne vulgaris: a double-blind trial. Acta Dermatovener 1980;60:337-340

[50] Michaelsson G, Luhlin L, Ljunghall K. A double-blind study of the effect of zinc and oxytetracycline in acne vulgaris. Br J Dermatol 1977;97:561-566

[51] Michaelsson G. Oral Zinc in acne. Acta Dermatovener 1980;89(suppl):87-93

[52] Dreno B, Amblard P, Agache SS, Litoux P. Low doses of zinc gluconate for inflammatory acne. Acta Derm Venerol 1989;69:541-43

[53] Michaelsson G. Decreased concentration of selenium in whole blood and plasma in acne vulgaris. Acta Derm Venerol 1999;70:92

[54] Michaelsson G, Edqvist L-E. Erythrocyte glutathione peroxidase activity in acne vulgaris and the effect of selenium and vitamin E treatment. Acta Derm Venerol 1984;64:9-14

[55] McCarthy M. High chromium yeast for acne? Med Hypoth 1984;14:307-310

[56] Ayres S, Mihan R. Acne vulgaris: therapy directed at pathophysiologic defects. Cutis 1981;28:41-42

[57] Open-Label Study of a Propietary Vitamin-Mineral-Herbal Nutritional Supplment in Mild to Moderate Acne Vulgaris. (Poster presentation) American Academy of Dermatology: Academy '05, July 2005 Chicago

[58] Morohashi M. Therapy of acne vulgaris with Kampoh drugs. Maruho Dermatol Sem 1984;43:17-22

[59] Higaki S, Haruki T, Morohashi M. The Clinical effect of Kampoh drugs to acne patients. Acta Dermatologica 1988;83:537-542

[60] Liu W, Shen D, Song P, Xu X. Clinical observation in 86 cases of acne vulgaris treated with compound olenlandis mixture. J Tradit Chin Med 2003;23:255-6

[61] Shuichi H, Kakamura M, Morohashi M, Hasegawa Y, Tamagishi T. Anti-lipase activity of Kampo formulations, Coptidis rhizoma and its alkaloids against Propionobacterium acnes. J Dermatol 1996;23:310-314

[62] Seki T, Morohashi M. Effect of some alkaloids, flavonoids and triterpenoids, contents of Japanese-Chinese traditional herbal medicines, on the lipogenesis of sebaceous gland. Skin Pharmacol 1993;6:56-60

[63] Lalla JK et al. Clinical Trials of Ayurvedic formulations in the treatment of acne vulgaris. J Ethnopharmacol 2001;78:99-102

[64] Paranjpe P, Kulkarni PH. Comparative efficacy of four Ayurvedic formulations in the treatment of acne vulgaris: a double-blind randomised placebo-controlled clinical evaluation. J Ethnopharmacol 1995;49:127-132

[65] Thappa DM, Dogra J. Nodulocystic acne: oral gugulipid versus tetracycline. J Dermatol 1994;21:729-731

[66] Dogra J, Aneja N, Saxena VN. Oral gugulipid in acne vulgaris management. Ind J Dermatol 1990;56:381-383

[67] Your mom. Daily reminder throughout your adolescence

[68] Guttman C. Acne myths still confuse patients. Dermatology Times 2005(May):44

[69] Mills OH, Kligman AM. Acne detergicans. Arch Dermatol 1975;111:65-8

[70] Fulghum DD, Catalano PM, Childers RC, Cullen SI, Engel MF. Arch Dermatol 1982;118:658-9

[71] Allen HB, LoPresti PJ. Acne vulgaris aggravated by sunlight. Cutis 1980;26:254-6

[72] Mills OH, Porte M, Kligman AM. Enhancement of comedogenic substances by ultraviolet radiation. Br J Dermatol 1978;98:145-50

[73] Chiu A, Chon SY, Kimball AB. The Response of skin disease to stress: Changes in the severity of acne vulgaris as affected by examination stress. Arch Dermatol 2003;139:897-900

[74] Sleep Loss Tied to Impaired Glucose Tolerance. Skin and Allergy News June 2005 page 51